Practitioner's Guide to Chakra Therapy

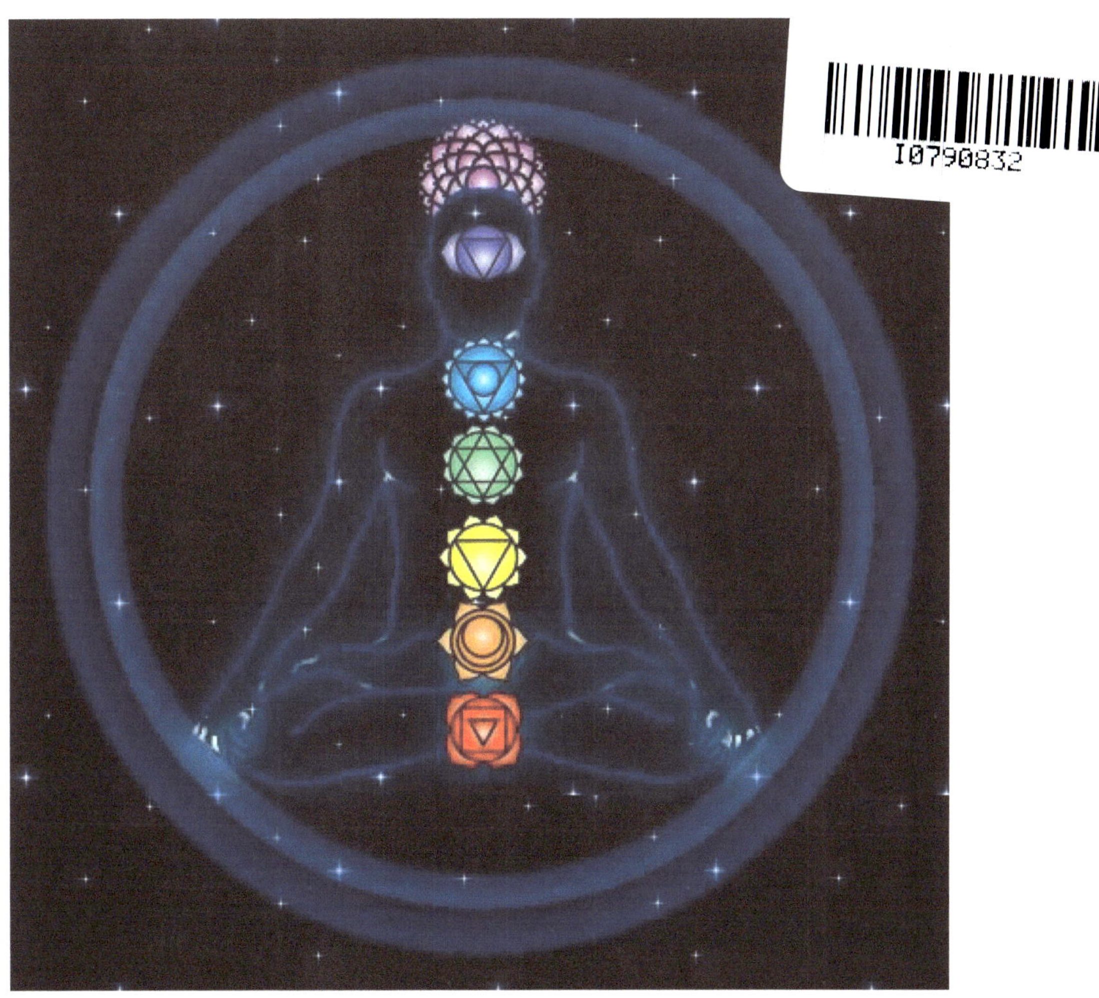

I0790832

Aruna Dawn
www.reikiraysinstitute.com
reikirays@yahoo.com

Copyright © 2017 Aruna Dawn for Reiki Rays Institute Press

All rights reserved. Except as permitted under U.S. Copyright Act of 1976, no part of this publication may be reproduced, distributed, or transmitted in any form or by any means, or stored in a database or retrieval system, without the prior written permission of the author.

Library of Congress Cataloging-in-Publication Data

ISBN-13: 978-1977580436

ISBN-10: 1977580432

Published in the United States of America
Reiki Rays Institute Press, Kansas USA

The information contained in this book are not intended to substitute competent medical advice. Those with health concerns should speak with their healthcare provider before making any treatment plan changes. Reiki Rays Institute, the author, and the publisher cannot be held responsible for reactions or side effects that may happen should the reader choose to follow the guidance shared in this manual.

First Edition

Welcome to Reiki Rays Institute's course in chakra therapy.

This book serves as a hard copy paper manual for the certified chakra therapy course offered by Reiki Rays Institute. If you have not already done so, to officially enroll and work towards that certification, please enroll by ordering our course online at
www.reikiraysinstitute.com/chakra.htm

There is no time limit to complete the course, and we are always just an email away.
Thank you for allowing us to share this information with you. Each person that joins us on our mission to share positive energy in the form of love, healing, and blessings helps make the world a safer, more peaceful place.

Warm Regards,

Aruna Dawn, President
reikirays@yahoo.com

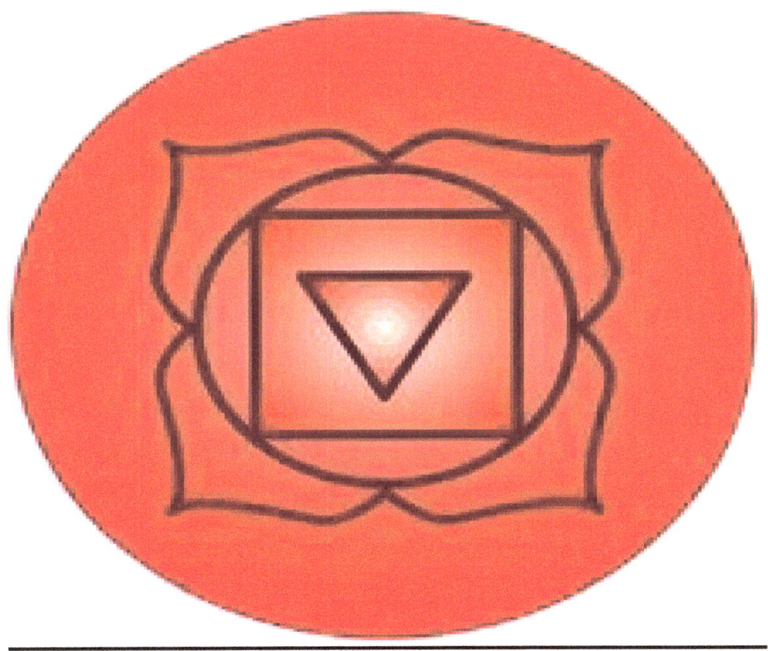

THE CHAKRA SYSTEM

Chakra is a Sanskrit word for "wheel of light". The chakra system consists of 7 main energy centers along the spine that are believed by many cultures to hold the key to health, happiness, and spiritual connectedness. Each chakra has a specific purpose, and if the energy of that chakra becomes disturbed, illness can take place.

There are seven musical notes that correspond to the seven colors of the rainbow, and these are related to the seven main chakras, which in turn correspond to different areas of the endocrine gland system. A series of tone sessions facilitates the rebalancing of each receiver back into an elevated level of etheric radiance.

The Base or **Root Chakra** is associated with the color red. This chakra is the grounding force that allows us to connect to the earth energies and empower our beings. Physical Location - base of the spine. In Sanskrit, the root is called Muladhara.

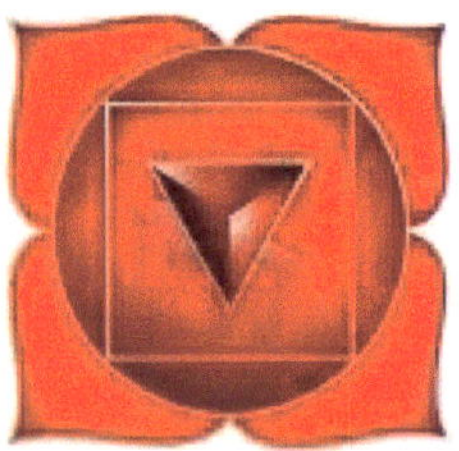

- Purposes - kinesthetic feelings, movement

- Spiritual Lesson - material world lessons

- Physical dysfunctions- lower back pain, sciatica, varicose veins, intestinal issues, depression, lowered immunity.

- Mental/Emotional Issues - survival, self esteem, social order, security, family

- Information stored in base chakra - familial beliefs, superstitions, loyalty, instincts, physical pleasure or pain, touch

- Area of Body Governed -spinal column, kidneys, legs, feet, rectum, immune system

- Gemstones – jasper, garnet, ruby, black tourmaline, any red stone or stone with grounding properties

- Essences – Rosemary, patchouli, cedar

- Musical note- C

- Age of Maturity- conception to age 7

The **Sacral Chakra** is associated with the color orange or red-orange. This chakra often offers us the opportunity to lessen our "control issues" and find a balance in our lives, teaching us to recognize that acceptance and rejection are not the only options in our relationships. The process of making changes in our life stream through our personal choices is a product of second chakra energy. Physical Location - lower abdomen to the navel. Its Sanskrit name is svadhisthana.

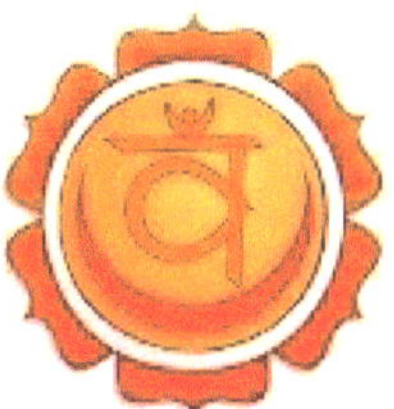

- Purposes - emotional connection

- Spiritual Lesson - creativity, manifestation, learning to "let go"

- Physical dysfunctions - low back pain, ob/gyn problems, pelvic pain, libido, urinary problems

- Mental/Emotional Issues - blame, guilt, money, sex, power, control, creativity, morality

- Information stored in sacral chakra - duality, magnetism, controlling patterns, emotional feelings (joy, anger, fear)

- Area of Body Governed - sexual organs, stomach, upper intestines, liver, gallbladder, kidney, pancreas, adrenal glands, spleen, middle spine

- Gemstones – carnelian, aragonite, tangerine quartz, any orange stone.

- Essences – vanilla, ylang ylang

- Musical note- D

- Age of Maturity- 7-14

The **Solar Plexus Chakra** is associated with the color yellow. This is the area which defines our "self-esteem". The personality that develops during puberty is housed in this chakra, otherwise known as the "EGO". Anyone experiencing dysfunction of the third chakra is having difficulty obtaining or maintaining his/her own "personal power". This intuitive chakra is where we get our "gut instincts" that signal us to do or not to do something. Strong self-esteem is a required for developing intuitive skills. Its Sanskrit name is Manipura.

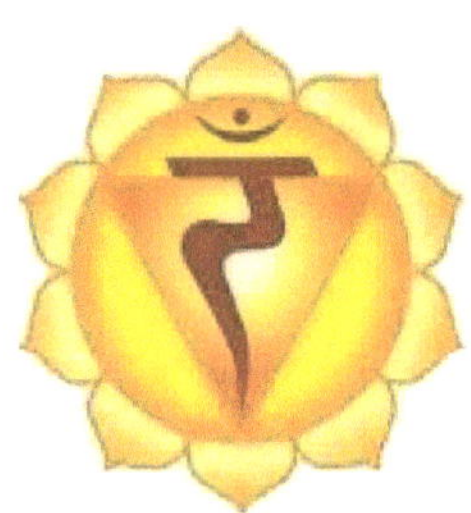

- Physical Location – center of stomach

- Purposes - mental understanding of emotional life

- Spiritual Lesson - acceptance of your place in the life stream. (self-love)

- Physical dysfunctions - stomach ulcers, tumors, diabetes, pancreatitis, indigestion, anorexia/bulimia, hepatitis, cirrhosis, adrenal imbalances, arthritis.

- Mental/Emotional Issues - self esteem, fear of rejection, oversensitivity to criticism, self-image fears, fears of our secrets being found out, indecisiveness

- Information stored in solar plexus chakra - personal power, personality, consciousness of self within the universe (sense of belonging), knowing

- Area of Body Governed - upper abdomen, rib cage, liver, gallbladder, middle spine, spleen, kidneys, adrenals, small intestines, stomach.

- Gemstones - citrine, Golden/imperial Topaz, amber, any golden or yellow stone

- Flower Essences – Peppermint, cinnamon, ginger

- Musical Note- E

- Age of Maturity- 14-21

The **Heart Chakra** is associated with the color green or pink. This love center of our human energy system is often the focus in bringing about a healing Physical illnesses brought about by heartbreak require that an emotional healing occur along with the physical healing. Physical Location -center of chest. Its Sanskrit name is Anahata.

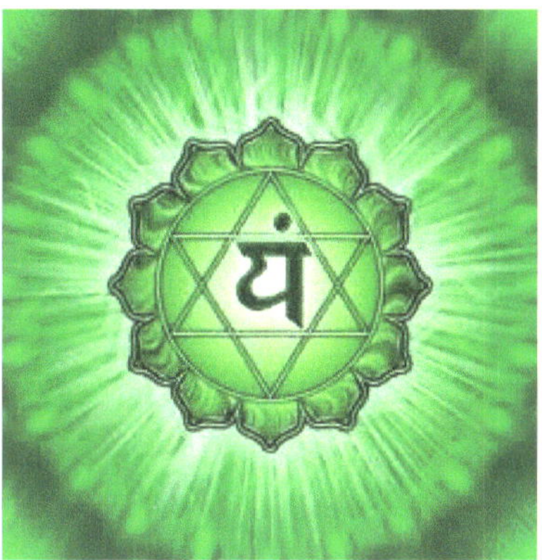

- Purposes - emotional empowerment

- Spiritual Lesson - forgiveness, unconditional love, letting go, trust, compassion

- Physical dysfunctions - heart conditions, asthma, lung & breast cancers, pneumonia, upper back, shoulder problems

- Mental/Emotional Issues - love, compassion, confidence, inspiration, hope, despair, hate, envy, fear, jealousy, anger, generosity

- Information stored in heart chakra - connections or "heart strings" to those whom we love

- Area of Body Governed - heart, circulatory system, blood, lungs, rib cage, diaphragm, thymus, breasts, esophagus, shoulders, arms, hands

- Gemstones –rose quartz, emerald, morganite, aventurine, any green or heart healing stone

- Essences – rose, jasmine, lavender

- Musical Note- F

- Age of Maturity- 28-35

The **Throat Chakra** is associated with the color sky blue. This chakra is our will center. The healthfulness of the fifth chakra is in relation to how honestly one expresses himself/herself. Lying violates the body and spirit. We speak our choices with our voices (throats). All choices we make in our lives have consequences on an energetic level. Even choosing not to make a choice such as in repressing our anger (not speaking out) may manifest into laryngitis. Physical Location - throat, neck region. Its Sanskrit name is Visuddha.

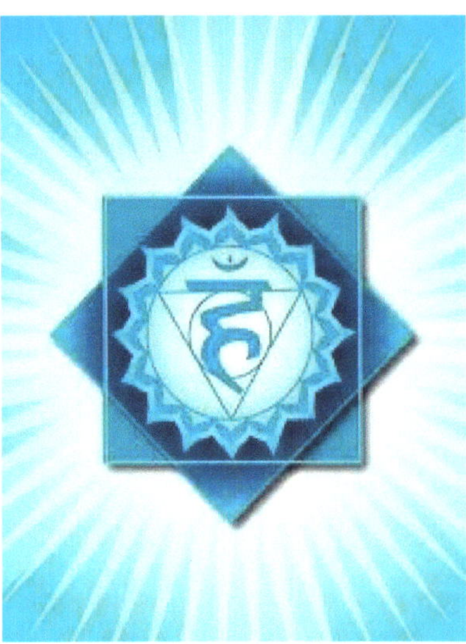

- Purposes - learning to take responsibility for one's own needs

- Spiritual Lesson - confession, surrender personal will over to divine will, faith, truthfulness over deceit

- Physical dysfunctions - sore throat, mouth ulcers, scoliosis, swollen glands, thyroid problems, laryngitis, voice problems, gum or tooth problems, TMJ

- Mental/Emotional Issues - personal expression, creativity, addiction, criticism, faith, decision making (choices), will, lack of authority

- Information stored in throat chakra - self-knowledge, truth, attitudes, hearing, taste, smell

- Area of Body Governed - throat, thyroid, trachea, neck vertebrae, mouth, teeth, gums, esophagus, parathyroid

- <u>Gemstones</u> – blue lace agate, blue chalcedony, angelite, any light blue stone

- <u>Essences</u> – lemon, eucalyptus, spearmint.

- Musical Note- G

- Age of Maturity- 35-42

The **Brow Chakra/3rd Eye** is associated with the color indigo. It is also often referred to as the "third eye" or the "mind center". It is our avenue to wisdom - learning from our experiences and putting them in perspective. Our ability to separate reality from fantasy or delusions is in connection with the healthfulness of this chakra. Achieving the art of detachment beyond "small mindedness" is accomplished through developing impersonal intuitive reasoning. It is through an open brow chakra that visual images are received. Its Sanskrit name is Anja.

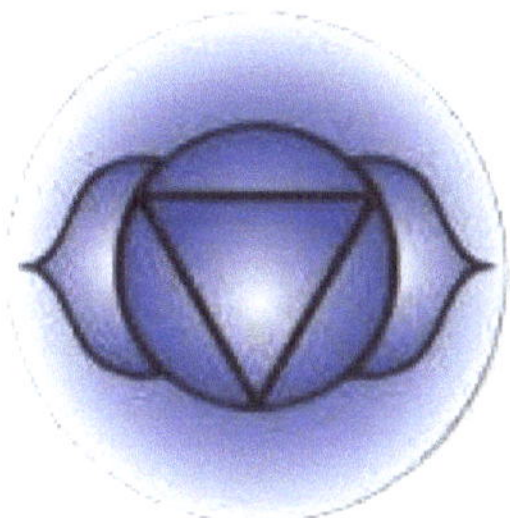

- Physical Location - center of the forehead

- Purposes - action of ideas, insight, mind development

- Spiritual Lesson - understanding, detachment, keeping an open mind, faith in a higher power/God

- Physical dysfunctions - brain tumors, strokes, blindness, deafness, seizures, learning disabilities, spinal dysfunctions, panic, delusions

- Mental/Emotional Issues - fear of truth, discipline, judgment, evaluation, emotional intelligence, concept of reality, confusion

- Information stored in brow chakra - seeing clear picture (symbolic or literal), wisdom, intuition, mental facilities, intellect

- Area of Body Governed - brain, neurological system, eyes, ears, nose, pituitary, pineal glands

- Gemstones – charoite, amethyst, Sugilite, sodalite, any indigo stone

- Essences – lemongrass, mugwort, cocoa

- Musical Note- A

- Age of Maturity- 35-42

The **Crown Chakra** is associated with the color indigo or clear/white. We use the seventh chakra as a tool to communicate with our spiritual nature. This chakra is often pictured as a lotus flower opening to allow spiritual awakening in an individual. Its Sanskrit name is Sahasrara.

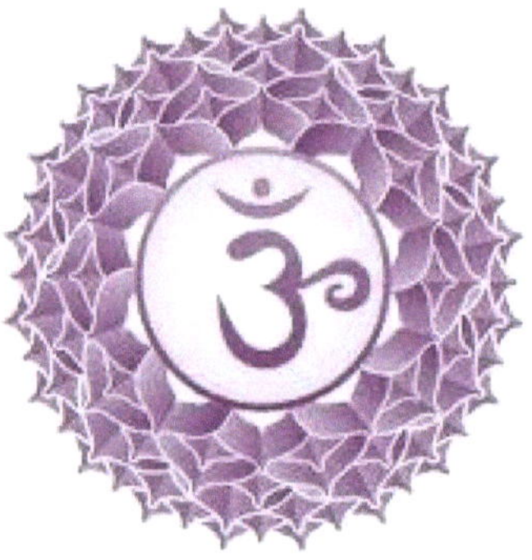

- Physical Location - top of head

- Purposes - intuitive knowing, connection to one's spirituality, integration of the whole

- Spiritual Lesson - spirituality, living in the NOW

- Physical dysfunctions - mystical depression, diseases of the muscular system, skeletal system and the skin, chronic exhaustion not associated with physical ailments, sensitivity to light, sound, environment

- Mental/Emotional Issues - discovery of the divine, lack of purpose, loss of meaning or identity, trust, selflessness, humanitarianism.

- Information stored in crown chakra - concept of the whole

- Area of Body Governed - top center of the head, midline above the ears

- Gemstones - danburite, Herkimer diamond, amethyst, quartz, any purple or clear stone

- Essences – frankincense, anise, white lotus

- Musical Note- B

- Age of Maturity-42+, based on the other chakra development. Some never have a full maturation of the crown and this is based on their spiritual and personal growth.

<u>Progress Test #1</u>

(For your own notes and not to be mailed in)

What does chakra mean?

Name the seven chakras

What musical notes correspond to each chakra?

List a gemstone that is associated with each chakra

Chakra Correspondences Chart

Chakra	Location	Function	Color
First	Feet to base of spine	Grounding	Red
Second	Genital area	Sexuality	Orange
Third	Abdominal area	Personal power	Yellow
Fourth	Heart	Love, healing	Green
Fifth	Ear, nose, throat	Communication	Light or aqua Blue
Sixth	Brow	Inner wisdom	Dark blue, indigo
Seventh	Crown of head	Oneness	Purple or clear

CHAKRA THERAPY WITH GEMSTONES

Simply place a gemstone or strand of gemstones on a Chakra and keep them there from 3-25 minutes. Here are the stones that are recommended on each chakra:

1. Root/Base: Red jasper, red tiger's eye, ruby, any red stone

2. Sacral: Carnelian, tangerine quartz, topaz, any orange stone

3. Solar Plexus Chakra: Citrine, tiger's eye, amber, any golden stone

4. Heart: Rose Quartz, malachite, aventurine, any green stone

5. Throat: Larimar, blue lace agate, turquoise, any blue stone

6. Brow/Third Eye: sodalite, sugilite, iolite, any indigo/ deep bluestone

7. Crown: Amethyst, charoite, lepidolite, any purple stone

Chakras & Essential Oils Associations

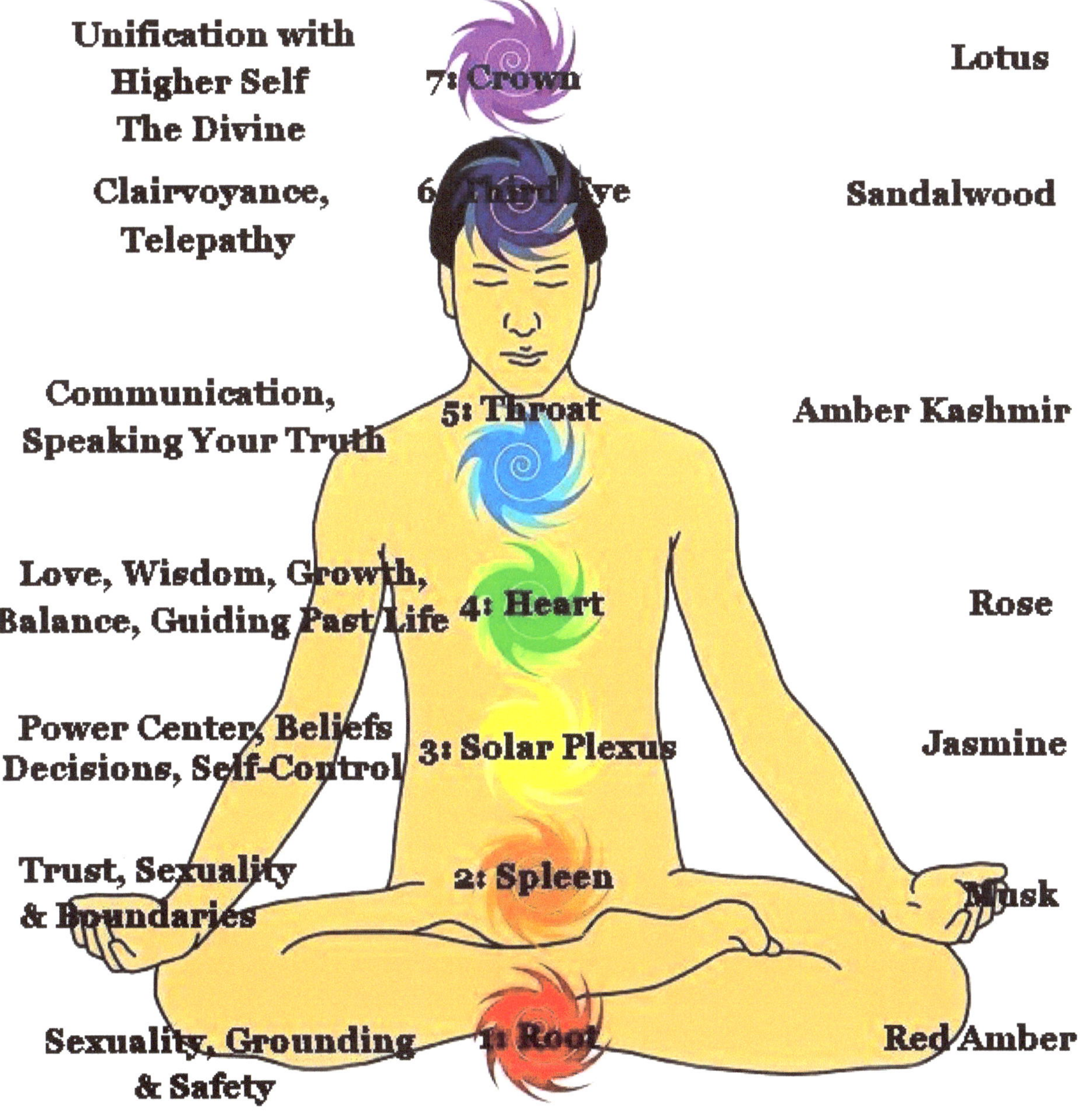

13

Essential oils and blends of the oils that appear below, can be anointed on the body, anointed on the stones, diffused in the air, or applied on the soles of the feet for further energetic assistance. Please DO NOT USE OILS ON PETS, as there have been mixed veterinary studies that indicate it can overwhelm and overtax the kidneys and other organs. Never consume oils, even if they sound innocent enough like peppermint or lemon, unless the bottle clearly indicates it is safe for consumption. If you cannot locate the oils listed in our picture, feel free to substitute:

Root — patchouli, pine, or any tree based oil

2nd — geranium, cinnamon, or cassia

3rd — orange, lemon, lime, any citrus

4th — ylang ylang, jasmine, lavender, or any floral

5th — eucalyptus, rosemary, peppermint, or any menthol type oil

6th — lemongrass or sage

7th — frankincense, myrrh, sandalwood, or unscented oil blessed for Divine work

<u>The Human Chakra System Chart</u>

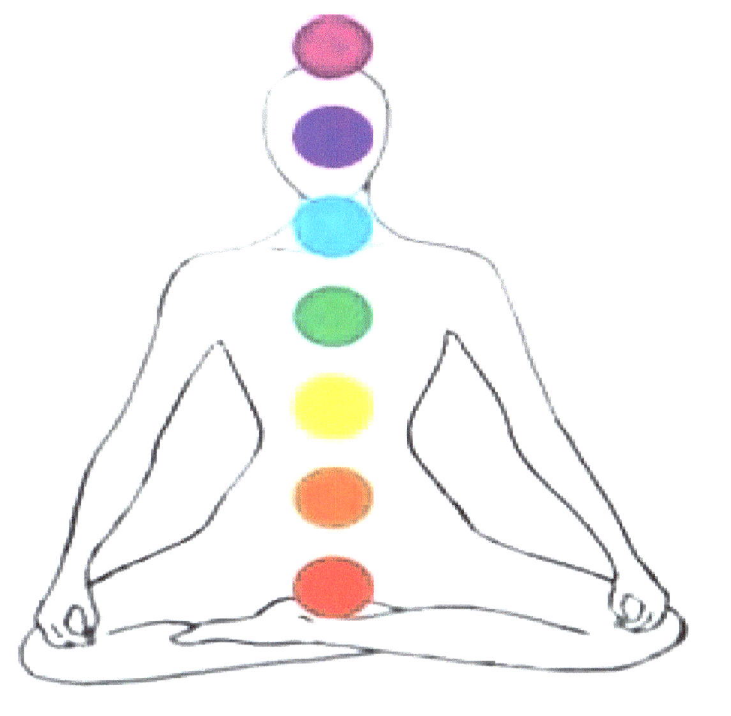

<u>Dog Chakra System</u>

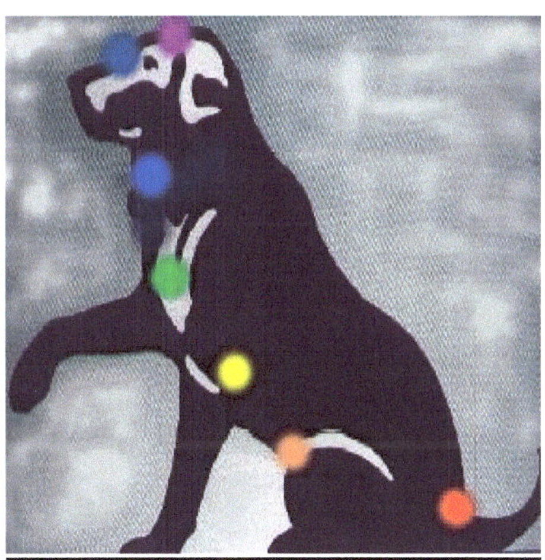

Cat Chakra System

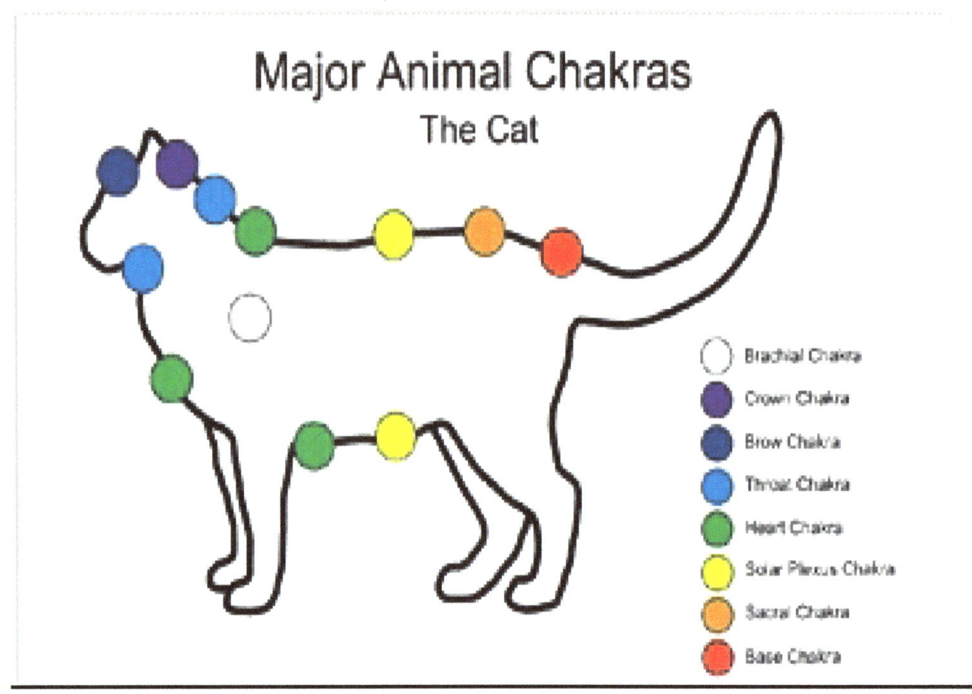

Horse Chakra System

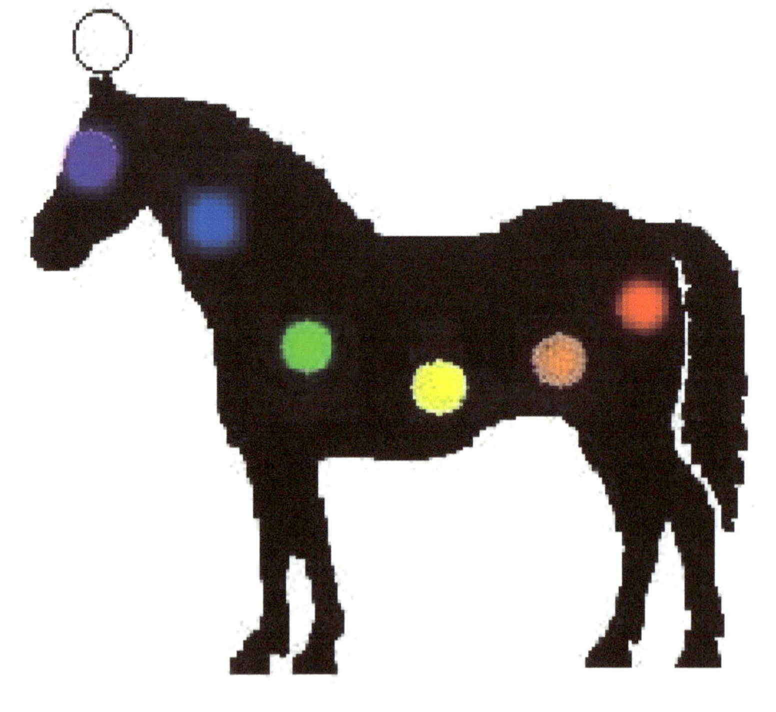

FOOD THERAPY

The chakras resonate with specific foods that carry a vibration that heals and stabilizes them. When you wish to bring healing to a specific chakra, you may want to change the emphasis of your normal diet to include more of these food types.

ROOT CHAKRA

Meats, chicken, and grains such as wheat, oats, and brown rice are beneficial. Red fruit such as apples, tomatoes, and red berries all carry the red energy of the Root Chakra. Also useful are national or religious dishes that convey community identity. Any favorite food from childhood can also stimulate the Root Chakra and is a reminder of a time the world was safe and carefree.

SACRAL CHAKRA

Fish, other seafood, algae, oranges, citrus, melons, sweet potatoes, squash, pumpkins, and carrots are all good for this center. Dishes that are sensuous to eat and stimulate the memory of good times are also beneficial.

SOLAR PLEXUS CHAKRA

Chicken, eggs, sunflower and olive oils, honey, molasses, pineapple, lemons, grapefruit, and brown rice are all good for this chakra and easy to digest. Food that is good against liver stagnation, such as green vegetables, and foods that aid digestion serve this chakra.

HEART CHAKRA

Heart of lamb, chicken, and beef are good for the Heart Chakra, as are small amounts of wine and sprouts, other greens, and low-fat cottage cheese. Foods rich in omega fatty acids such as salmon are good for the heart, too. The heart needs good nutrition to be strong. It does well with good food that increases circulation.

THROAT CHAKRA

The Throat Chakra likes food that is easy to swallow. It does not like mucous-producing foods such as chocolate, dairy products, or excess sweets. When the throat is sore, lemon and honey are soothing.

BROW CHAKRA

In ancient times salmon, tea, and almonds were thought to be good for the brain. Salmon was the fish of wisdom to the ancient Celts. Aristotle said six almonds and tea were good for the brain. Eating lightly keeps the mind clear. Food that is fresh, free of additives, and high in protein is excellent for the Brow Chakra.

CROWN CHAKRA

Fasting is the "food" of the spirit. Occasional fasts at changes of the seasons purify the blood and open the spirit to changing earth rhythms and cycles. Fasting helps us be grateful for the abundance available to us that we are able to choose from.

	PHYSICAL BODY	EMOTIONAL BODY	MENTAL BODY
ROOT CHAKRA	ADRENALS: the fight-or-flight function of the kidneys is activated.	Aggression, anger, violence, jealousy.	Attitudes of separation, exclusivity, territory, belonging, your right to your own space.
SACRAL CHAKRA	OVARIES/TESTES: the reproductive organs, which control sexual development.	Pleasure, feeling good, deservedness, joy/feeling bad, envious, not caring for your physical body.	Attitudes of being and having enough, knowing that you deserve the life you say you want, enjoyment and well-being, delighting in good health, disdain for suffering.
SOLAR PLEXUS CHAKRA	PANCREAS: the organ that processes sugar. It also controls the digestion of food.	Self-worth, confidence, power, clear choices for selfhood.	Attitudes of being well with yourself and knowing your worth, linking into your personal power, which comes from an affirmed sense of selfhood.
HEART CHAKRA	THYMUS: building a strong immunity from pain and disease.	Being capable of love and compassion for self and others.	Attitudes of happiness, joy, and delight, knowing what and who make your heart sing, embracing life.
THROAT CHAKRA	THYROID: controls metabolism and affects physical and mental development.	Releasing feelings through expressing yourself. This includes crying, shouting, laughing, and saying that you are not happy, comfortable, or pleased.	Having a clear sense that expressing your truth is your key to individuality. Speaking the truth, not gossiping, lying, exaggerating.
BROW CHAKRA	PITUITARY: influences metabolism, growth, and other hormones, including those connected with giving birth.	Giving yourself permission to experience your feelings, whatever they are. Choosing when it is appropriate to express how you feel.	Attitudes that are self-confirming, accepting, inclusive. Developing understanding for your own limitations and those of others, cultivating forgiveness and gratitude.
CROWN CHAKRA	PINEAL: produces melatonin and regulates our body clock.	Wanting to cultivate bliss and surrender to what is.	Developing holistic and universal principles of acceptance, respect, and knowing that we never do anything without the help of a higher source.

The Archetypes of the Chakras

Each chakra is associated with a healthy archetype, and a dysfunctional archetype. Sometimes the easiest way to see what chakra or chakras need attention is to focus on personality traits that come through.

The first chakra relates to security, so if a baby feels neglected, 'the victim' develops, as they cannot meet their own needs. The solution is then, 'the earth mother,' where one nurtures one's self.

The second chakra is about personal responsibility, self-expression, abundance and believing we deserve to enjoy life. Out of balance, people will see themselves as a 'martyr.' The remedy here is 'the sovereign,' who looks for the best in things.

The third chakra is about our relationship with ourselves, self-esteem, and personal power. The healthy archetype is 'the spiritual warrior,' balancing inner-strength with belief in a divine guiding force. Its opposite is 'the drudge,' who depends on others for approval, projecting onto others the power they wished they possessed (which they do, if only they could acknowledge it).

The fourth chakra balances the love of others and ourselves. 'The lover' is healthy as they truly own themselves and radiate love. Its counterpart is 'the performer,' who looks outside for the love they seek, fooling themselves that someone external will heal their wounds.

The fifth chakra is associated with communication and self-expression. 'The communicator' is the healthy version, as opposed to 'the masked self,' who hides behind comedy or unrealistic positivity to cover up feeling no-one will listen. This creates a self-fulfilling prophecy, where if 'the masked self' revealed their truth, they would become the communicator, who is listened to.

Chakra six is about perceiving and knowing, represented by the third eye. When this is balanced, 'the psychic' is the archetype, where the person trusts their instincts, which they weigh with theory. The opposite is 'the rationalist,' who is stuck in intellectualizing and following rules, causing increasing limitations.

The seventh chakra is related to wisdom, consciousness, and spiritual connection. 'The guru' has given up attachment, accepts personal limitations and is aware that all things are possible. 'The egocentric' focuses on self-determination and control, leading to materialism, which is eventually found meaningless, putting 'the egocentric' into crisis, where they can become 'the guru.'

The solution to these chakra challenges is in the analysis, where once one understands their behaviors and motivators, they are able to make more conscious, healthy choices.

Chakra Toning

A powerful technique to resonate and balance your chakras using vowel sounds. This is a good exercise to do every day, and is a great introduction to exploring the harmonics naturally present in the vowels.

Vowels carry the "information energy" of speech, whereas consonants act to break up the energy flow. In ancient Sanskrit, Hebrew, Chinese, etc., the vowel sounds are considered to be sacred. In other words, the vowel sounds carry the intention and focus.

Start by sitting comfortably in a chair or on a cushion on the floor. Try to keep your spine as straight as possible, which allows the energy to flow in your body more freely – it may help to imagine your head is suspended from above by a fine cord, letting your body hang below it naturally.

Make these sounds in a gentle voice – don't strain. Focus your energy and intent for balancing and energizing each chakra before toning. To find the correct pitch for a particular chakra, scan up and down feeling in your body for a resonance (apart from the throat where it will always resonate). The pitch will change according to the person, mood, diet, activities, emotional states, etc. on a daily basis. There is no set frequency.

The first chakra (Root) – located at the base of the spine. Tone seven times with the deepest "UUH", as in "cup", a very low guttural sound just gently riding on the breath. Stay comfortable with the sound – don't force it. (Red).

Second chakra (Sacral) – located about 2-3 inches below the navel. Tone seven times using a higher pitched but still deep "OOO", as in "you". (Orange).

Third chakra (Solar Plexus) – located above the navel. Tone seven times using a higher pitched "OH", as in "go". (Yellow).

Fourth chakra (Heart) – located in the centre of the chest. Tone seven times using a higher pitched "AH", as in "ma". This is the sound that embodies compassion. (Green).

Fifth chakra (Throat) – Tone seven times using a higher pitched "EYE", as in "my". (Blue).

Sixth chakra (Third Eye) – located in the middle of the forehead slightly above the eyes. Tone seven times, using a still higher "AYE", as in "say". (Indigo).

Seventh (Crown) – Tone seven times using the highest pitched "EEE" sound, as in "me", you can comfortably make. (Violet or white).

Chakras and Astrology

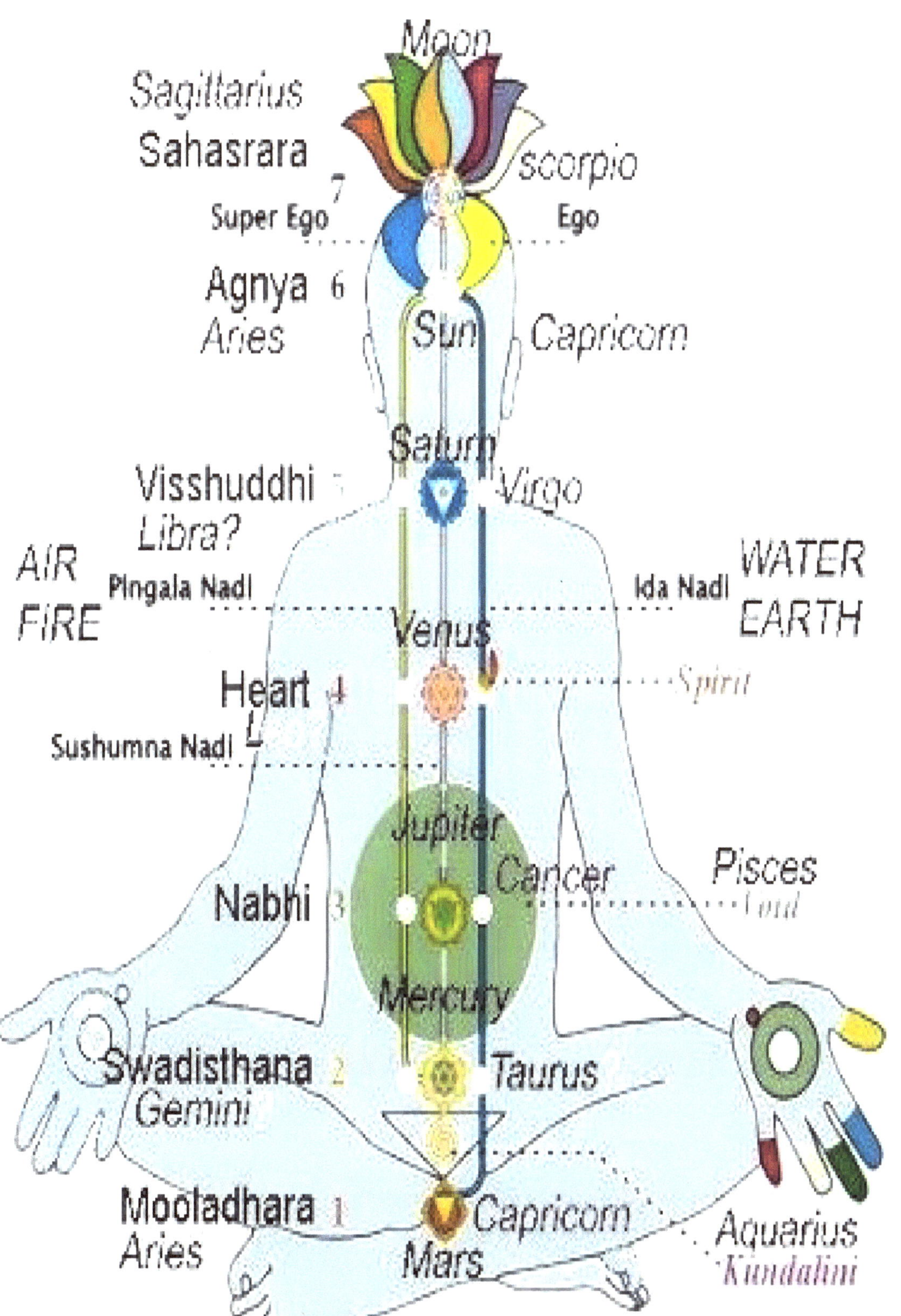

BIJA MANTRAS FOR CHAKRA MEDITATION
For Purification, Protection, and Light of the Divine Mother[†]

Purification Balance	**Protection** Perfection	Light Expansion
Crown/Sahasrara Soundless Sound **AUM**	**OM AIM HRIM SHRIM** **KLIM SOU HU OM**	**AUM**
Third Eye/Ajna **OM NAMAHA**[*]	**OM KRIM NAMAHA**	**SHRIM**
Throat/Vishuddha **OM HAM NAMAHA**	**OM SOU HU NAMAHA**	**SOU HU**
Heart/Anahata **OM YAM NAMAHA**	**OM AIM HRIM KLIM** **CHAMUNDAYE VICHE**	**KLIM**
Solar Plexus/Manipura **OM RAM NAMAHA**	**OM SHRIM NAMAHA**	**HRIM**
Seat-of-the-Soul/Svadhishthana **OM VAM NAMAHA**	**OM HRIM NAMAHA**	**GLOUM**
Base-of-the-Spine/Muladhara **OM AIM NAMAHA**	**OM AIM NAMAHA**	**AIM**

Yoga Poses for Chakra Balancing

For those who practice yoga, the following poses may help with chakra alignment:

Muladhara: Mula (root) adhara (support) – Located at the tip of the coccyx and the pelvic floor, this chakra is associated with physical identity, survival, stability, and instinctual nature. Psychologically it relates to fear, feeling lost, and anger. Physically it corresponds to fatigue, poor sleep, lower-back pain, immune disorders, and obesity.

To strengthen muladhara, we build strength, physically grounding the body with the stability of the earth so we can be rooted, self-aware, courageous, and fearless.

Asanas: Mountain Pose, Warrior Pose, Standing Forward Bends

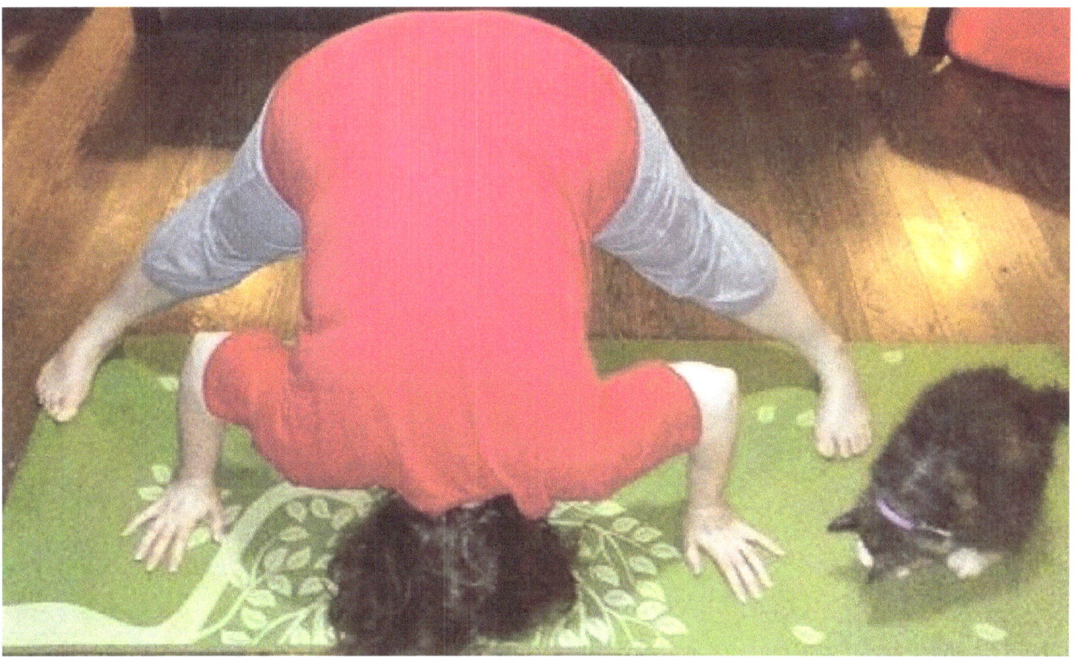

Wide legged standing forward bend, and my cat Bebe, doing her own version

Svadhisthana: The Sacral Chakra- Seat of Vital Force – Located between the sacrum and pubic bone, including the genitals, svadhisthana corresponds with the center of gravity of the body. This chakra relates to the cultivation of the emotional and sensual self. It is the home of the reproductive organs, the kidneys, the hips, and the sacrum.

Fluidity, sensual pleasure, and dance, as well as physical and emotional expression, are all rooted in this second chakra. It is psychologically connected to power and control issues, morality, obsession, guilt, blame, and addiction. The power released in the physical world with this chakra is not to be trifled with. This chakra often relates to emotional identity, desire, procreation, self-love (especially physical), and relationships. It relates to health issues associated with libido, sciatica, lower-back pain, vertigo, menstrual issues, and hormonal imbalances.

When balanced, svadhisthana produces a balanced, vital, sexually uninhibited, prosperous, satisfied way of being.

Asanas: Triangle pose, Wide-Stance Seated Position, Seated Bound Angle Pose

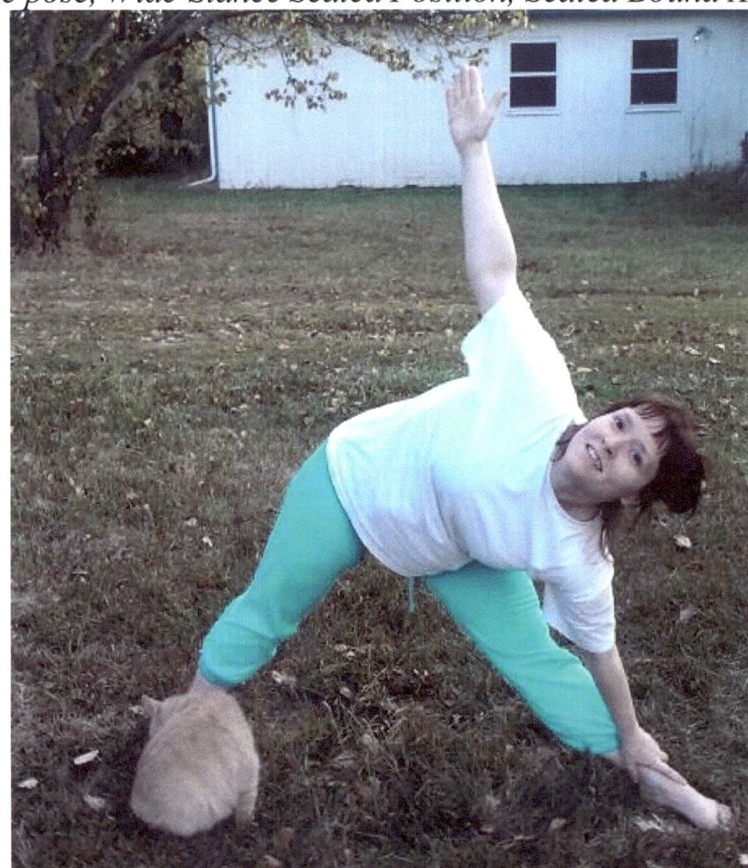

Triangle Pose with my cat, RayRay

Manipura: The Solar Plexus Chakra- City of Jewels – Located at the solar plexus, manipura is a central point of transformation in the body. In these alchemical practices, when we really want to change, we engender fire (manipura's element) and burn away our former selves to allow for a new self to emerge. Jewels also function as prisms, bending light to change the look of reality, thereby reminding us that reality is shaped by perception.

Some of the organs associated with manipura include the stomach, liver, gallbladder, midspine, and small intestines. This chakra can help you deal with psychological issues like low self-esteem, timidity, depression, fear of rejection, perfectionism, anger, indecisiveness, and rage.

When manipura is balanced, one feels confident, clear, decisive, productive, and focused, and one's digestion is excellent.

Asanas: Half-twist, Boat Pose, Backbends.

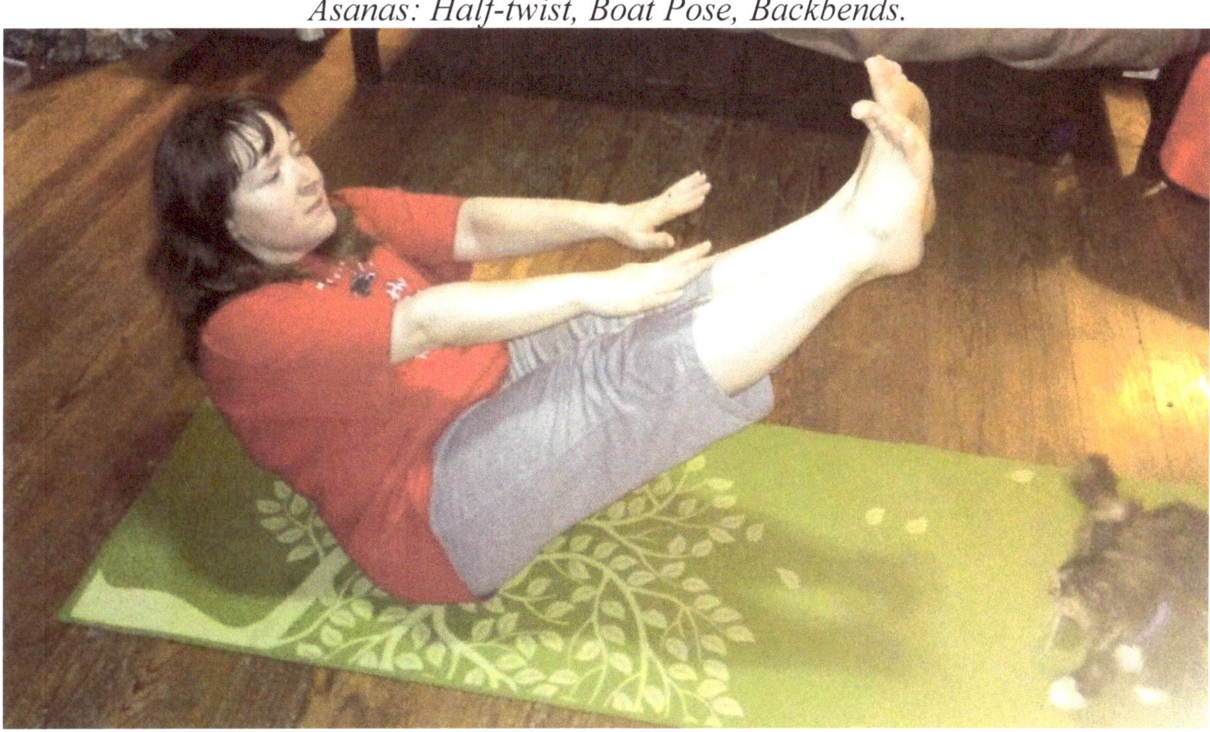

Boat Bose

Anahata – The Heart Chakra- Anahata literally means "unbeaten." It is the heart chakra and the center point in the chakra system, standing between the three lower earthly chakras and the three celestial chakras above. Through the heart chakra we harmonize heaven and earth, finding the dynamic balance between spiritual practice and living in the earthly realm. It is my belief that this chakra holds the power to transcend pain and suffering.

At the core of this chakra is love, and love is the unifying healing force that links us all together. One of the best ways to strengthen the heart chakra is to offer it openly to the world.

Asanas: Eagle Pose, Cow Pose, Cobra, Wheel Pose, Chest-opening poses

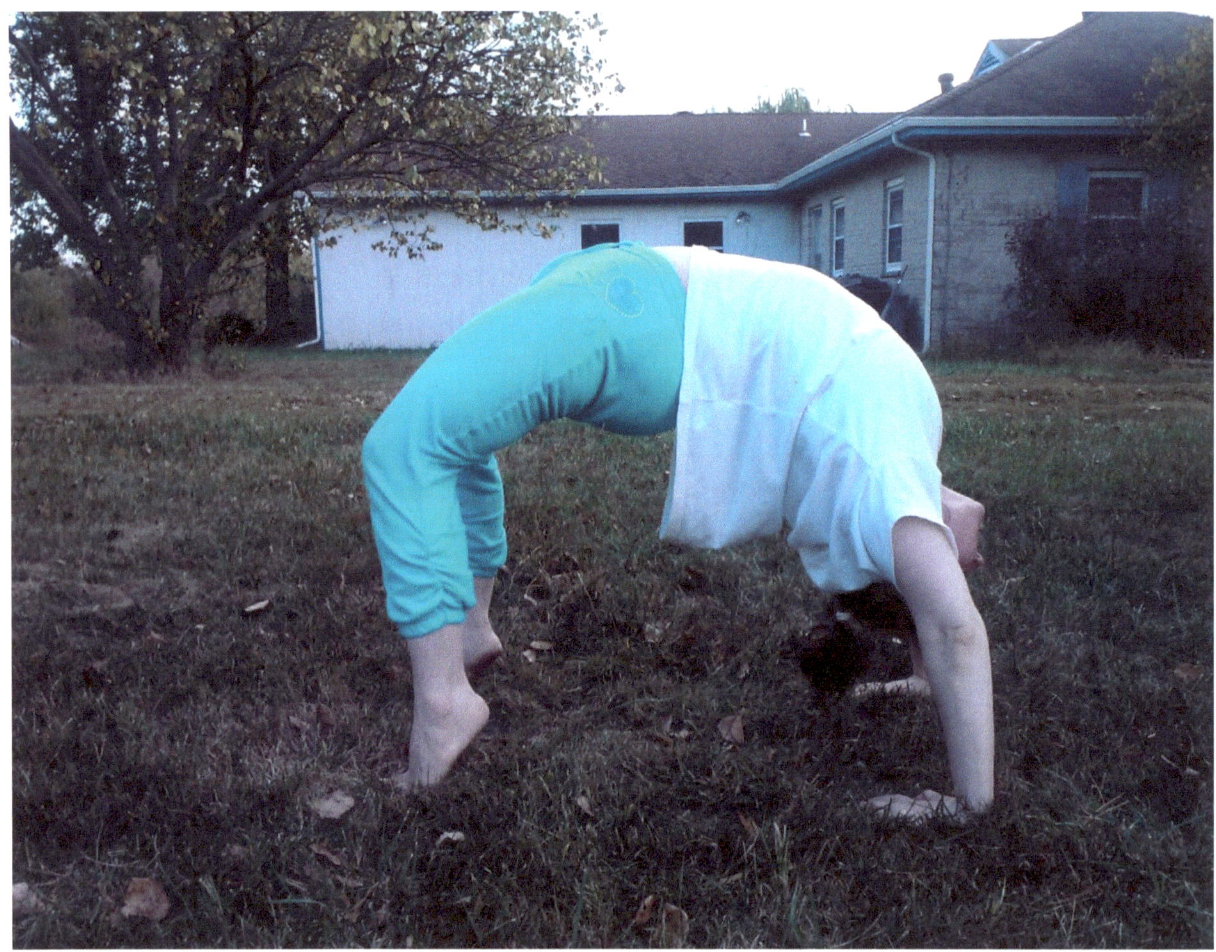

Wheel Pose

Visuddha: The Throat Chakra- Purification – Unlike the lower chakras, visuddha is focused on the spiritual and metaphysical path. Located at the throat, this chakra connects the spiritual and physical plane through the vibration of sound.

The reading of poems and prayers and chanting are all excellent ways to express the positive nature of this chakra. The throat, thyroid, and parathyroid glands are always associated with visuddha, and they are often healed through communication and creativity.

Asanas: Fish Pose, Lion Pose, Shoulder Stand

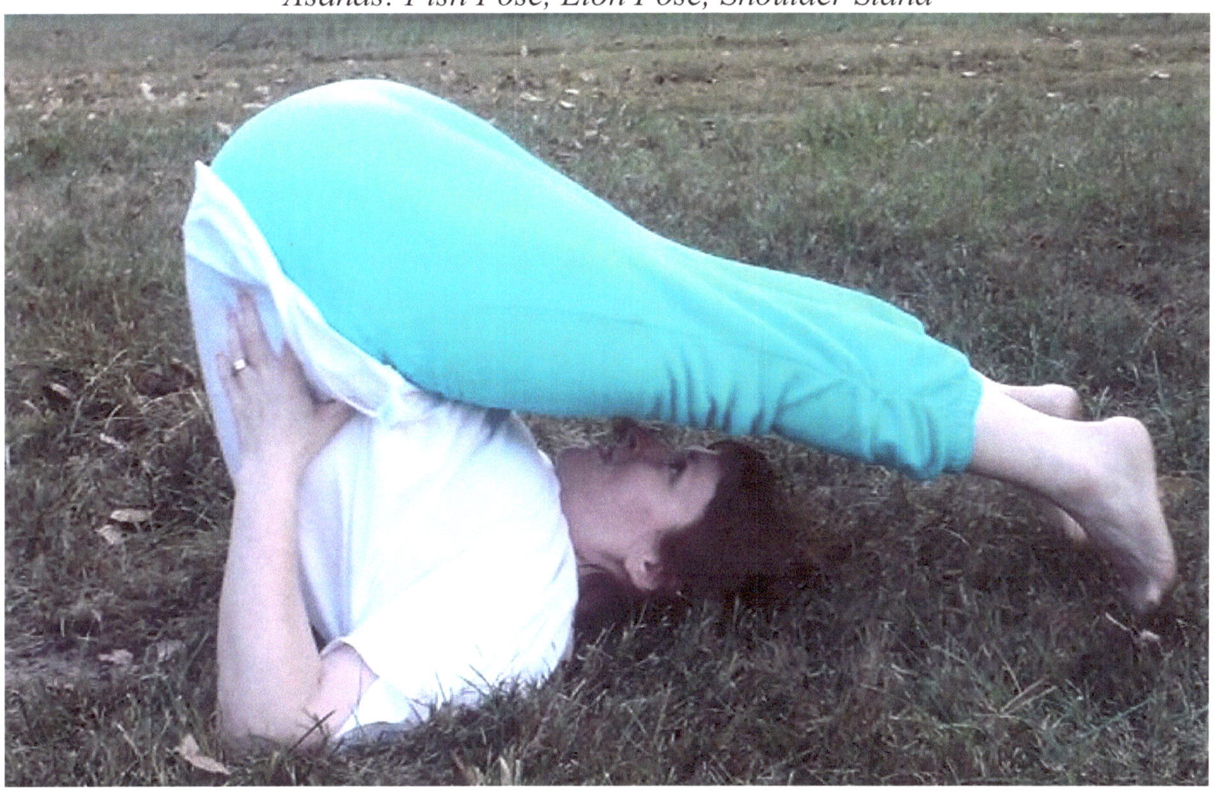

Fully Extended Shoulder Stand

Ajna: The Third Eye Chakra – Located between the two eyebrows, ajna is related to inner vision. This chakra sits in the acupuncture point often translated as "calm spirit," and provides us with the unique gift of being able to link our sight with our crown chakra to access the greater collective consciousness. This is the chakra we use to scan our body and energetic field for disturbances.

This chakra requires rooting in the earth element through the breath in order not to overactivate it. Dysfunction of this chakra can lead to headaches, nightmares, eyestrain, and learning disabilities. When balanced, this chakra produces a deep, clear calm and is capable of creating reality from thought.

Asanas: Breath work, meditation, Child's Pose, Yoga Nidra

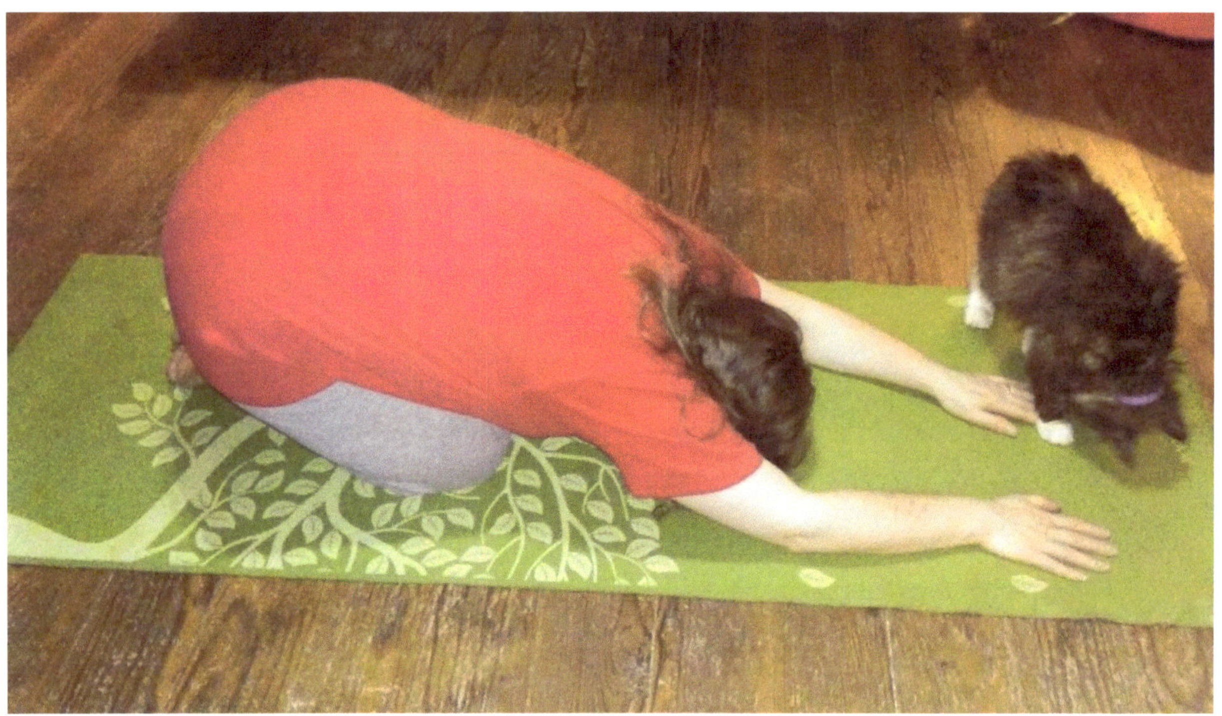

Child's Pose- Bebe doing her own version

Sahasrara: The Crown Chakra- One-Thousand-Petaled Lotus – The lotus represents the infinite creation and destruction of all things. Located at the crown of the head, sahasrara allows you to directly receive celestial information and to connect with deities and other energy forces available to you.

This chakra, when open, can collapse time and space and allow the future and past to be available to you simultaneously. Often misinterpreted as seeing the future, a deep connection with sahasrara allows you to see everything in the now.

Asanas: Tree Pose, Eagle Pose, Seated Meditation

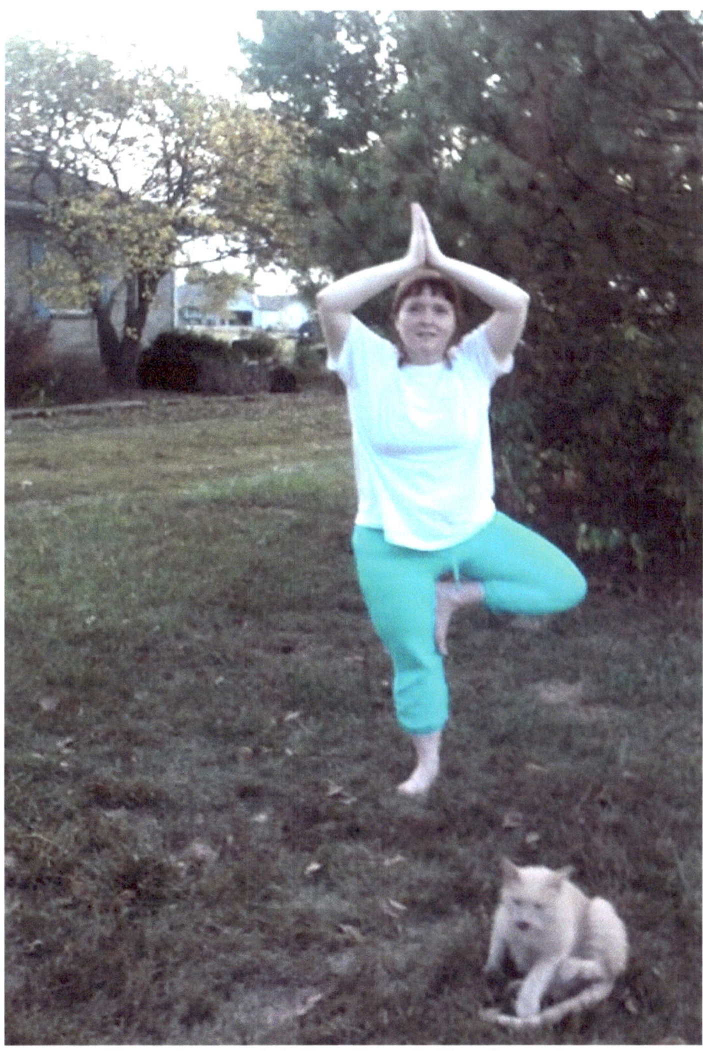

Tree Pose with RayRay following along

Preparation for a Session

If you are already skilled in Reiki or any other holistic art, feel free to do whatever preparations you are comfortable with before the session. Balancing can be done with the client standing, sitting, or laying down, so decide what will be of most comfort for them.

I highly recommend that you purify your working space with incense, oils, and/or meditation/prayer. Feel free to invite your guides/angels/God to assist you with this work. If nothing else, make sure that you visualize a protective white light around you and your client for the work ahead. Either silently or aloud declare that your intent in balancing the chakras is for the highest good for all parties involved. If you know you will be working on animals, I suggest as noted previously that oils not be applied to them directly or where they can potentially consume/lick the oils. Diffusing in the air does not seem to be an issue provided the pet is not accidentally sprayed directly.

Ask your client to decide what position they are going to be most comfortable in. They need not remove any clothing. It may be advised that they remove their shoes or jewelry, but absolutely no nudity is required or necessary for the balancing. I suggest that for animals that you cover your table with a cloth that is used solely for pet work for sanitary purposes, and do know that animals are prone to want to walk around and leave the area during sessions, which is fine. You will need to modify your session to allow them for mini breaks, but do return to the session after just a few minutes.

If you will be treating someone distantly, it may help if you have a photo or can visualize what they look like- otherwise meditation on their name, address, and what you do know about them will be important for the procedure to take affect.

Please view your manual to become familiar with the chakras, their properties, locations, etc. When you are confident that you are familiar with this material, it will then be time for you to begin to treat yourself or others. Gather your stones and mists. You need not use these items,

but their colors and properties are especially helpful for beginners. There are special incenses, oils, and other chakra products available to assist you. You may contact me for more info on how to obtain these optional items.

Preliminaries to a Session

For chakra healing in person the stones can be placed

1. ***Upon the subject.***
   Be extra careful when placing stones in the breast and genital regions.

2. ***Below the subject.***
   Under the table is equally effective, especially if you are going to be doing other holistic therapies.

3. ***Around him or her.***
   Many practitioners prefer to run the stones along the left side of the body.

For Distance Sessions

You can use a substitute, sometimes called a proxy, to stand in for the client who is at a distance from you. A photograph of the client is a great substitute, however, if no photo is available, writing down their name and using that is good also. Once you do this regularly, it will be much easier, and you are likely to develop your own unique routine. When I was new to visualization, I often used a stuffed animal or pillow as a substitute.

Simply modify the directions below, and while doing them, either hold their picture, go into meditation, or if you have visualization abilities, simply see in your mind's eye their chakras and intuitively feel what is needed to bring them into harmony.

Balancing the Chakras

Start first with the root chakra. Hover your hands over the region WITHOUT TOUCHING THE AREA. Place your stone alongside of or on top of the region if you like. If working remotely, or if your client does not want stones place on their body, use the chakra photo in the manual and place a stone on the region. A corresponding essential oil may be rubbed onto the stone prior to placement. Now visualize the chakra opening up like a door or window, and see the color red flowing from the chakra. You may also sense that it is blocked or even overactive. Use your mind's eye to make the region glow a beautiful deep red. When you see this, state out loud or to yourself a mantra something like "I PURIFY, ENERGIZE, AND BALANCE THE ROOT CHAKRA NOW". Now take your right hand and make 3 counterclockwise circles over the chakra, then shake out your hand. Repeat until you feel the energy is balanced. Then repeat using the left hand, this time using a clockwise rotation.

Next go to the sacral chakra. Hover your hands over the region WITHOUT TOUCHING THE AREA. Place your sacral stone alongside of or on top of the region if you like. If working remotely, or if your client does not want stones place on their body, use the chakra photo sheet enclosed in the manual above and place a stone on the region. A corresponding essential oil may be rubbed onto the stone prior to placement. Now visualize the chakra opening up like a door or window, and see the color orange flowing from the chakra. You may also sense that it is blocked or even overactive. Use your mind's eye to make the region glow a beautiful deep orange. When you see this, state out loud or to yourself something like "I PURIFY, ENERGIZE, AND BALANCE THE SACRAL CHAKRA NOW". Now take your right hand and make 3 counter-clockwise circles over the chakra, then shake out your hand. Repeat until you feel the energy is balanced. Then repeat using the left hand, this time using a clockwise rotation.

Next go to the solar plexus chakra. Hover your hands over the region WITHOUT TOUCHING THE AREA. Place your solar plexus stone alongside of or on top of the region if you like. If working remotely, or if your client does not want stones place on their body, use the chakra sheet enclosed and place a stone on the region. A corresponding essential oil may be rubbed onto the stone prior to placement. Now visualize the chakra opening up like a door or window, and see the color yellow flowing from the chakra. You may also sense that it is blocked or even overactive. Use your mind's eye to make the region glow a beautiful deep golden yellow. When you see this, state out loud or to yourself something like "I PURIFY, ENERGIZE, AND BALANCE THE SOLAR PLEXUS CHAKRA NOW". Now take your right hand and make 3 counterclockwise circles over the chakra, then shake out your hand. Repeat until you feel the energy is balanced. Then repeat using the left hand, this time using a clockwise rotation.

Next go to the heart. Hover your hands over the region WITHOUT TOUCHING THE AREA. Place your heart stone alongside of or on top of the region if you like. If working remotely, or if your client does not want stones place on their body, use the chakra picture sheet enclosed and place a stone on the region. A corresponding essential oil may be rubbed onto the stone prior to placement. Now visualize the chakra opening up like a door or window, and see the color green flowing from the chakra. You may also sense that it is blocked or even overactive. Use your mind's eye to make the region glow a beautiful deep color. When you see this, state out loud or to yourself something like "I PURIFY, ENERGIZE, AND BALANCE THE HEART CHAKRA

NOW". Now take your right hand and make 3 counterclockwise circles over the chakra, then shake out your hand. Repeat until you feel the energy is balanced. Then repeat using the left hand, this time using a clockwise rotation.

Next go to the throat chakra. Hover your hands over the region WITHOUT TOUCHING THE AREA. Place your blue lace agate alongside of or on top of the region if you like. If working remotely, or if your client does not want stones place on their body, use the chakra grid sheet enclosed and place a stone on the region. Now visualize the chakra opening up like a door or window, and see the color blue flowing from the chakra. You may also sense that it is blocked or even overactive. Use your mind's eye to make the region glow a beautiful deep blue. When you see this, state out loud or to yourself something like "I PURIFY, ENERGIZE, AND BALANCE THE THROAT CHAKRA NOW". Now take your right hand and make 3 counterclockwise circles over the chakra, then shake out your hand. Repeat until you feel the energy is balanced. Then repeat using the left hand, this time using a clockwise rotation.

Next go to the third eye chakra. Hover your hands over the region WITHOUT TOUCHING THE AREA. Place your amethyst alongside of or on top of the region if you like. If working remotely, or if your client does not want stones place on their body, use the chakra picture enclosed and place a stone on the region. A corresponding essential oil may be rubbed onto the stone prior to placement. Now visualize the chakra opening up like a door or window, and see the color purple flowing from the chakra. You may also sense that it is blocked or even overactive. Use your mind's eye to make the region glow a beautiful deep purple. When you see this, state out loud or to yourself something like "I PURIFY, ENERGIZE, AND BALANCE THE THIRD EYE CHAKRA NOW". Now take your right hand and make 3 counterclockwise circles over the chakra, then shake out your hand. Repeat until you feel the energy is balanced. Then repeat using the left hand, this time using a clockwise rotation.

Next go to the crown chakra. Hover your hands over the region WITHOUT TOUCHING THE AREA. Place your quartz alongside of or on top of the region if you like. If working remotely, or if your client does not want stones place on their body, use the chakra grid sheet enclosed and place a stone on the region. A corresponding essential oil may be rubbed onto the stone prior to placement. Now visualize the chakra opening up like a door or window, and see the color white or silver flowing from the chakra. You may also sense that it is blocked or even overactive Use your mind's eye to make the region glow a beautiful clear light. When you see this, state out loud or to yourself something like "I PURIFY, ENERGIZE, AND BALANCE THE CROWN CHAKRA NOW". Now take your right hand and make 3 counterclockwise circles over the chakra, then shake out your hand. Repeat until you feel the energy is balanced. Then repeat using the left hand, this time using a clockwise rotation.

When complete, visualize all chakras glowing with their corresponding color. It is now time to balance the entire energy field. You can do this by sweeping over the client from head to toe with a feather, wand, or even just your hands. It is recommended to sweep the entire body 7 times- the number of layers to the aura as well as the number of chakras. It is now time to close the chakras.

Closing the Chakras

It is a basic rule of nature to close what you have opened. To do this, you work in the reverse pattern that you cleared the chakras. Since you started with the root, then you will work from the head down. Simply brush over each chakra, just as you did with the entire aura. Visualize closing them each in turn, like a door or window. When you have finished the root, go to the client's feet and visualize the grounding out of the energies through their feet. You can visualize tree roots or earth, or anything that helps you see the client grounded.

Progress Test #2

How do you plan to prepare for a chakra therapy session?

What will be your balancing affirmation?

Why do you sweep the body seven times after balancing the chakras?

Hand Chakras

Most people are familiar with the 7 chakras that run up the center of the body, but there are minor chakras as well, such as the hand chakras. Even though they are considered as secondary chakras, the energy centers located in the palm of our hands are powerful tools of perception and healing. Healers appreciate the quality of energy flowing through their hand chakras, but also anyone, with a little awareness of energy, can grasp the importance of these centers.

Where are the Hand Chakras?

Hands are the centers for multiple chakras. The primary chakras are located in the center of each palm. Others are said to be located at each joint, which make hands particularly useful channels for energy healing. The palm chakras are the focal point for the hand meridians.

Healers have differing views on how to classify the hand chakras; some see them as primary chakras, others consider them as concentrated energetic fields in charge of transmitting energy from other chakras. For instance, healing work often involves the hands as primary means to feel, give, and receive energy. Healers may channel energy through and from other chakras, such as the root chakra and earth energy, or heart chakra and love.

Function of the Hand Chakras

Just like the other chakras, the centers of energy location in your hands are what allow you to interact with the world on an energetic level. They allow healing energy to flow both in and out and are associated with the act of giving and receiving.

Healthy hand chakras manifest as openness, creativity and confidence as you move through the world. They are usually associated with the color red or gold, although their shade and radiance may vary depending on the type of channeled energy.

Signs that your hand chakras may be blocked include:

- Lack of creativity and inability to express yourself artistically
- Feeling closed off or numb
- Lack of connection with the world and with other people

Hand Chakras and Energy Healing

Open hand chakras are essential for energy healing. If they are blocked or imbalanced, energy flow from the healer will be weak or inconsistent. Reiki and other energy healing modalities use hand positions to help energy get where it is needed, but blocked hand chakras make that difficult.

For self-healing, the same problems arise. Blocked hand chakras create a closed system rather than an open one, preventing energy from flowing freely through your body and getting where it needs to go. In addition, chakra hand positions, or mudras, can help balance the major chakras in the body. Blocked hand chakras will prevent these mudras from being effective.

How to Open the Hand Chakras

There are several methods for opening your hand chakras. One of the simplest is simply holding your hands in water. If possible, use a natural body of water such as a stream or a lake, but a bowl of water will work. As you let your hands rest, imagine the water gently washing away any blockages you might have and replacing them with bright, flowing energy.

Another useful exercise comes from Reiki. To begin, hold your hands with your palms touching each other and gently rub them together. Imagine a glow forming in the palms of your hands. After a moment, slowly bring your hands a few inches apart, still imagining a glowing ball of energy emanating from your palms. Feel the energy. You may feel warmth or tingling as you play with this energy. Move your hands around a bit, letting the energy move and grow. Imagine it flowing from each palm. Finally, bring your palms back together and allow the energy to flow back into your body, healing and energizing you.

Creating art is also excellent for opening chakras. Using your hands will help get creative energy moving through them. Hands-on methods like sculpting are especially good.

Balancing chakras takes time and consistent practice, but these exercises can be done in a few minutes a day. Regular focus on the rest of the chakra system will also help with balancing your hand chakras. Using mudras or Reiki hand positions during your meditation will allow you to work on your hand chakras while healing and balancing other parts of your body.

Electro-Graph Chakra Reflexes

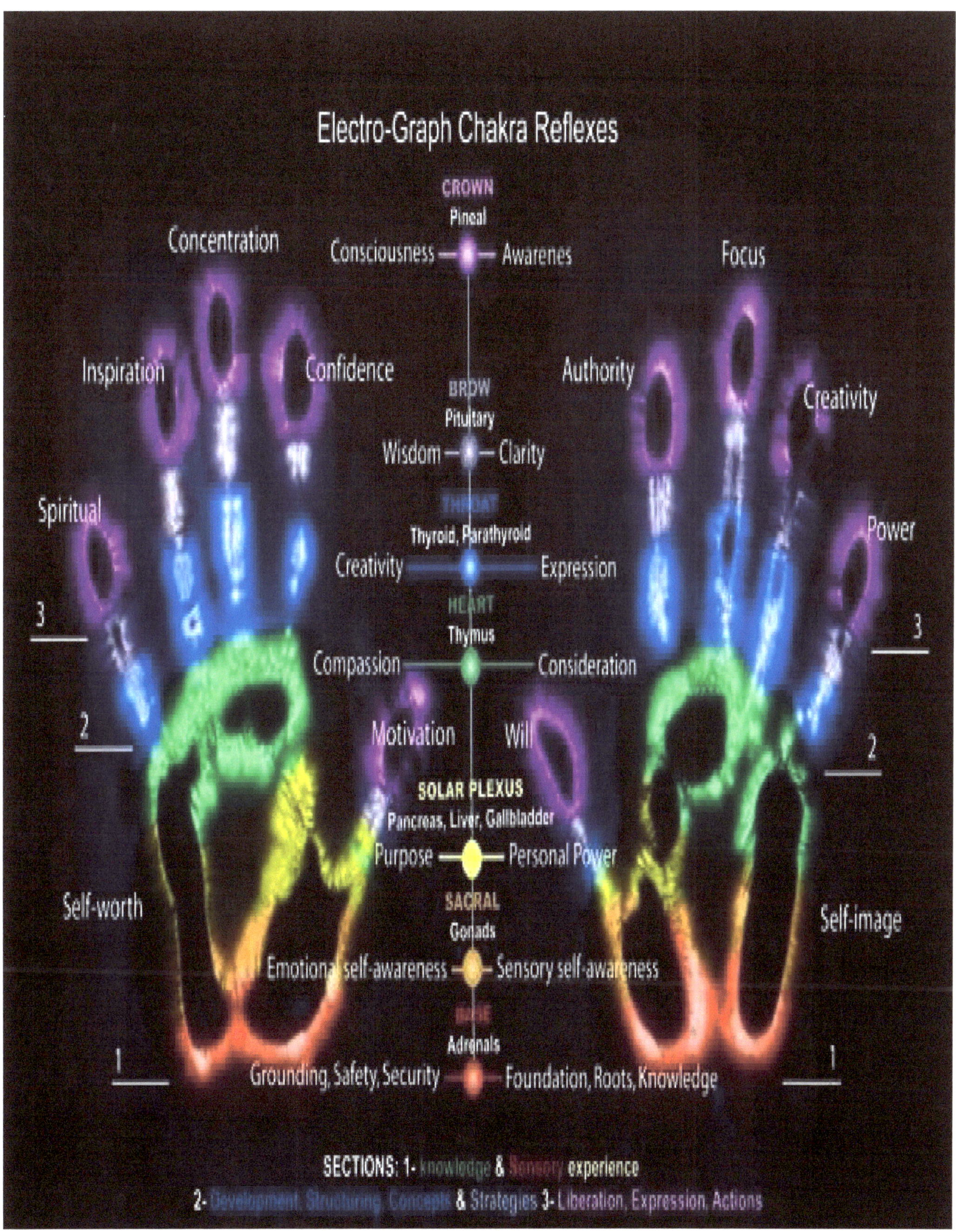

The Chakras of the Foot

In a physical sense, the foot chakra is actually a split energy center, with each half sitting in the ball of each foot. If you were to place your feet together, these centers would seem to combine and make a complete energy center. However, regardless of whether the feet are physically next to each other, these split-centers, on each foot, are always linked and are always complete.

Now, the foot chakra is an important center in that it is here that divine energy returns back to the Source. It is the last point at which the energy is a part of you. Traditional thinking places the base chakra as this grounding point; however, that reasoning is not entirely correct. You see! The base (or root) chakra's function is more than just a grounding center. It actually functions as an energy transformation point where divine energy gets slowed down so that it can pass into the Earth quickly and effortlessly. While the base chakra does the actual conversion, it does not do actual passing of the energy. Furthermore, the energy at the foot chakra remains elusive because this chakra, and the energy contained in it, has been nearly transformed into an Earth-based energy. Hence, as far as you can tell, the last place you perceive energy movement in the chakra system is at the base chakra, so you assume that no other major energy centers exist below it.

For example, if you could x-ray your energy centers and observe the energy stream as it enters from top, you would follow this energy as it slowly changed its form, as it passed from chakra to chakra. On this hypothetical x-ray, you would watch as the color shifted from the upper vibrations toward increasingly lower vibrations, as it passed from one chakra to the other. From the *base chakra* to the *foot chakra*, you would not see a corresponding shift in color or be able to distinguish it from the background color of the Earth itself. However, if you were to adjust this x-ray a bit and examine for a flow of energy, instead of a color shift, you would notice a concentrated stream of energy reaching down from the base chakra and going into the foot chakra, where it would then swirl around for a bit and pass on into the Earth and back to ALL-THAT-IS. This swirling at the foot chakra is important and is a result of the amount of blocked up energy that can't freely pass into the Earth, and it is here the next part of our discussion begins.

An ideally, fully-open foot chakra would have no swirling whatsoever in it. It would pass energy out as quickly as it entered. Here, I'm speaking of an indefectible case and only the most adept individuals (like a Master) possess a foot chakra free of all blockages. In a more realistic sense, though, an open foot chakra will have a slight swirling going on at all times. This kind of openness shows an individual that has no trouble keeping his focus on the mundane. It also shows that this person integrates well with earthly structures and energy systems. These people are usually very healthy as the earth-based energy can pass quickly out of the body's energy system and take most of the built-up negativity out of the system before it has a chance to do any harm and possibly manifest as an illness.

On the other hand, a closed foot chakra, where a great deal of swirling is going on, shows a person that is in a blocked-up state. The energy has no place to go, so it backs up and leaks out of the other (higher) centers and into the surrounding aura and atmosphere, where it is then absorbed by the Earth Plane. This leaking is very undesirable because energy that does not pass through the foot chakra and exits through the other centers cannot be used by the individual. This kind of leaking also carries away much positive energy and, as such, these people will often be tired, irritable, and unreasonable.

Also, with the foot chakra blocked, all the areas of well-being may get affected negatively. The individual poorly integrates with peers and loved ones and cannot understand other people's point of view. In an extreme case, such an individual will rebel against society and claim that everyone is after him and out to do him in. They become very fearful and may even resort to violence as a kind of defense mechanism to protect the little energy that they have that is still of use to them. Some types of destructive behaviors are believed to stem from an extensively blocked-up foot chakra.

Of course, in the above, I am talking about an extreme case. With a very ordinary type blockage, you would see a very mild form of these kinds of behaviors. Children, for example, often exhibit the mild symptoms of a blocked foot chakra. They are often self-centered and selfish with their possessions and with dealing with other children. In many children, the foot chakra is not fully developed, so it can't effectively pass energy out. Energy tends to back up in them quickly. In fact, you can notice this backing up in spurt patterns. The spurts are due to children holding on to their divine energy too long and then when the back-up becomes too intense, they force open up their foot chakra and release the energy out in one lump sum. This holding/releasing pattern is normal in children, because they have not learned how to fully ground themselves. Eventually, as the child's foot chakra develops, and they ground better, they become more giving and tolerant of themselves and others. These spurts of groundedness and being blocked will dissipate as the child enters adolescence and eventually will be almost non-existent. ALMOST is the key word here because, as I said, many adults have blocked foot chakras (many of these cases stem from childhood), and, thusly, they will take on very mild forms of these childish patterns.

The cure, of course, is to open up the foot chakra and get it to pass energy as quickly as possible out of the entire chakra system and into the Earth. Many illnesses and adverse behavior patterns can be alleviated just by doing work on this chakra. Opening up this chakra requires the same techniques as used in opening up the other centers. The only note to make here is that a pendulum reading is not apt to give you an accurate account of what is going on in the foot chakra, as the blocked, swirling energy can fool the pendulum and make it swing to indicate and fully open condition, when, in fact, the center is closed up.

A better way to determine if the foot chakra is blocked is to have the patient lie down on his/her back and put his/her feet upright with a 3 to 6 inch space between the feet. Next you need to place your hand just above the energy field of the foot chakra. This will be somewhere between 3 to 12 inches above the tops of the toes, centered over the gap in the feet. At this point, you want to take a temperature reading, using the palms of your hands as a thermometer. A very warm energy reading will indicate much swirling of energy and a blocked center. A very hot reading indicates a completely blocked center. A nice cool reading, with a faint tingling sensation in the palm of the hand, indicates an open center that is satisfactorily passing energy out of it. Here, of course, I recommend you feel what a good, clear center is like before you can tell what a blocked center feels like. Very quickly, you will develop a natural affinity for the way it feels when your hands are near this energy center.

If you are able to see the aura, you can observe for a blocked foot chakra. (With the word 'fine' here we are referring to being able to distinguish between the Earth's background energy field and that of the grounded energy passing out of the chakra system.) With this technique, you should direct your attention to between the feet and look for dark swirling, wispy, like streaks. A good clear foot chakra will show only one or two of these swirls. A blocked one will have more. A fully blocked foot chakra will be seen as a solid darkness that just permeates between the feet (you may not need to see fine aura to pick up on this one).

People tend to get a blocked foot chakra when life gets a bit too much for them. The increase in mundane activity backs-up energy in the foot chakra because the individual is not used to clearing this increased amount of energy flow. Quickly, a sense of fear or anticipation can pervade, as the other higher centers begin to leak energy out into the aura. People experiencing the onslaught of this condition will report an increase in sensitivity all over the body. They may become very emotional or even extremely intellectual, depending on their core makeup. Exercise can help here to alleviate this condition, temporarily, but eventually this energy center will have to be unblocked to permanently alter the condition. The other fix is to return to previous levels of mundane activity, which is undesirable because, if the individual is experiencing a growth in activity, it is likely that the person is ready to handle things on a more increased level.

Now, normally, this energy center will learn to open up on its own, when an increase in activity comes about, and it then passes the expanded energy flow out, returning the individual to status-quo, after a short period of discomfort. But, in some cases, possibly because of fear or because of not wanting to let go of old patterns and ways, this natural opening-up process does not occur and the individual gets forced to take a step back, thereby retarding their own growth. A trained energy practitioner can unblock this chakra very easily and see the results in the patient's life almost instantly. Many people who engage in intense spiritual development will experience this cycle of the foot chakra blocking up and then unblocking. They often feel like a yo-yo being pulled up to ecstasy one moment and then being gripped by fear of the unknown another. Again, the simple cure is to unblock this chakra.

To unblock this chakra conventional healing techniques will work. I will not be covering standard healing practices in this chapter, but, for those people that are not familiar with how to do this kind of healing or for those people reading that just want to be able to clear their own center, I have a procedure that will work quite nicely, under normal conditions and for normal blockages.

Get a standard clear drinking glass and fill it with two or three table spoons of sea salt. Fill the glass with water and mix up the salt and water until no sea salt remains. Now lie down on the floor on your back or sit in a meditation position and put the glass near or against the balls of your feet. The idea is to immerse the solution in the center of the Foot Chakra's energy field. Now, relax for three minutes or so. The sea salt solution will begin to pull any energy blocks out of the center. Now, after several minutes, sit upright, if you were on your back. And use your hand, and, in a swirling motion, hover it above the glass of sea-salt solution and above the energy field of your foot. This swirling distance of your hand should be no more than 6 inches above the tops of your toes. Continue to swirl this energy around for another minute, to coax the last of the blocks out of the chakra and into the sea salt solution. The procedure is complete! Now pick up the glass and yourself. Throw away the salt-water solution and wash the glass thoroughly.

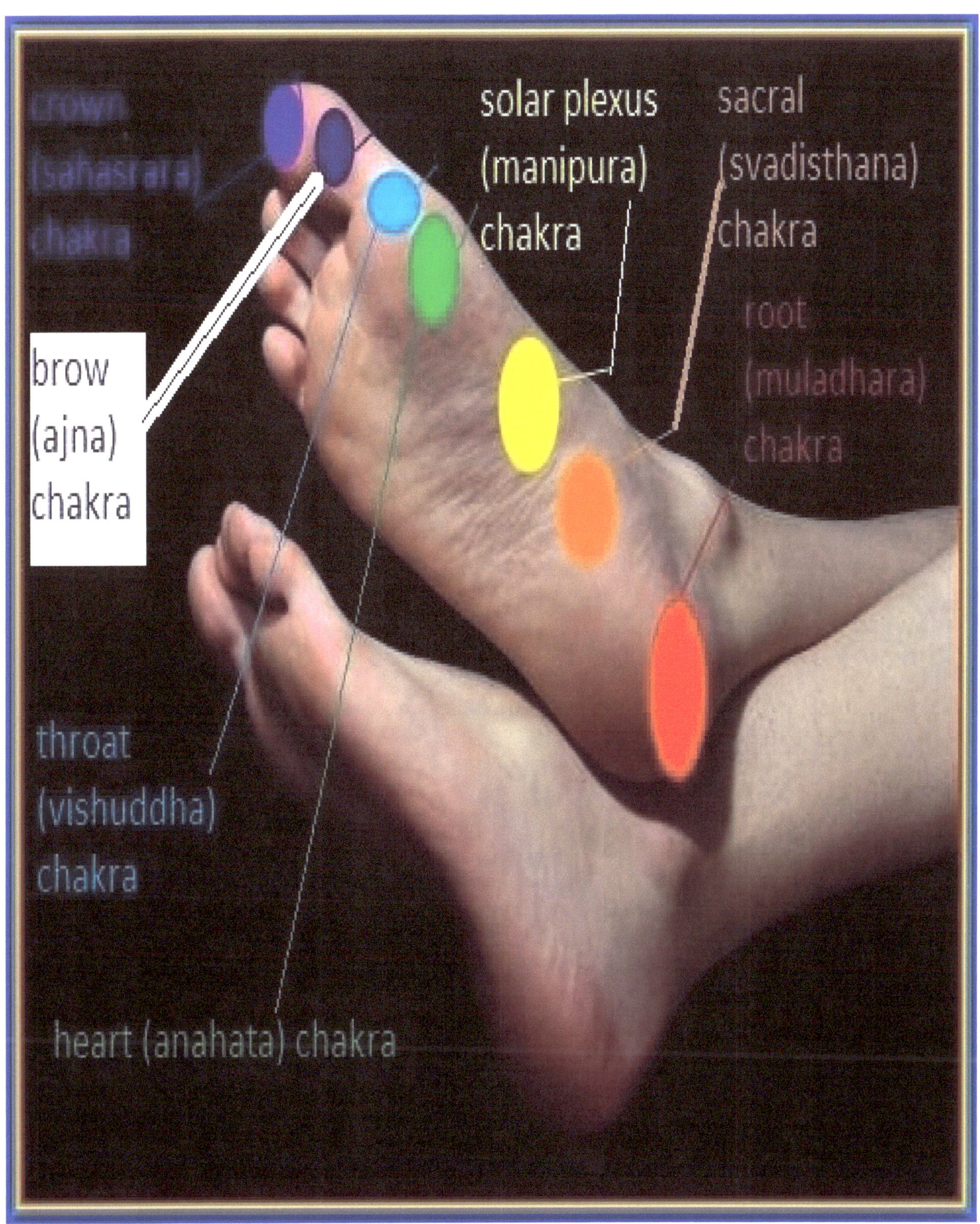

crown (sahasrara) chakra
brow (ajna) chakra
solar plexus (manipura) chakra
sacral (svadisthana) chakra
root (muladhara) chakra
throat (vishuddha) chakra
heart (anahata) chakra

Client/Practitioner Relationship

It is very important to create clear boundaries and rules for your practice, even if you have no plans to work professionally. If you are adding these skills to an already established holistic or medical healing practice, you will of course need to abide by the rules and regulations of your industry and region.

If you are working with friends and family, make sure you approach this work with the same level of seriousness and professionalism you would with a professional client. Since this is about energies, you will reap the results of the energy you put into the session, and you owe it to all clients, regardless of their closeness to you, to represent the session with the utmost respect.

Code of Conduct

1. Abide by a vow of confidentiality. Any information that is discussed within the context of a session is confidential between the client and the Practitioner.

2. Provide a comfortable area for classes and work to provide an empowering and supportive environment for students.

3. Always treat clients with the utmost respect and honor.

4. Provide a brief oral or written description of what happens during a session and what to expect before a client's initial session.

5. Be respectful of all other's views and paths.

6. Educate clients on the value of the system and explain that sessions do not guarantee a cure, nor are they a substitute for qualified medical or professional care. Chakra Therapy is one part of an integrated healing or wellness program.

7. Suggest a consultation or referral to qualified licensed professionals (medical doctor, licensed therapist, etc.) when appropriate.

8. NEVER diagnose or prescribe. Never suggest that the client change prescribed treatment or interfere with treatment of a licensed health care provider.

9. Never ask clients to disrobe (unless in the context of a licensed massage therapy session). Be sensitive to the boundary needs of individual clients. Do not touch the genital area or breasts. Practice hands off healing of these areas if treatment is needed.

10. Be actively working on your own healing so as to embody and fully express the core of everything that you do.

Progress Test #3

Prepare for yourself a code of ethics for your practice and post in your workspace.

Exercise 1- Feeling Subtle Energies

This is not as hard as it sounds. You will attempt to feel the energy field of a person. Rub your hands together for a minute or so, then place them together in 'prayer" position. Slowly separate them, very, very gradually. The key is to see if you can detect a magnetic sensation between them as you bring them close together, without touching.

What sensations did you feel? Please turn this in, or email your results, for evaluation.

Part 2—working with another's chakra energy field

Get into a focused state of mind, then rub your hands together and scan the other person's body, concentrating on the chakra regions. It may be easier to start off working around the head, neck, and shoulders or a place where you know the individual has had surgery, injury, or pain. See if you can detect temperature differences.

Try the above with at least one other person, this time doing it over various parts of their body if possible and not just their hands.   What did you feel? Record your sensations below. Please turn this in, or email your results, for evaluation.

You may find that this is easier with some people than others. You can even try this with pets and observe their reactions.

Prepare yourself to do a chakra session and warm up your hands by rubbing them. Hover your hand near any chakra (again the crown is often easiest for these practices but do not limit yourself to the crown) and after putting your hands in position, close your eyes part of the way, or look out of only the corner of your eye. Do you detect any color, heat, or movement/vibration?

Relax and give it a few minutes. Try this on every chakra on the person or pet. You can even try this on yourself by looking at your reflection in the mirror. This is a difficult exercise and do not worry if you do not have immediate results! Record your experience below.

<u>***CASE STUDY #1 SELF CHAKRA CLEARING***</u>

YOUR NAME____

Any current health complaints? YES   NO

Please
expain:____
____
____
____

What Chakra(s) do these ailments correspond to?
____
____
____

What did you feel during the session?
____
____
____
____

How did you feel after the session?
____
____
____

Did you have any problems or questions while performing this session?   YES   NO
If yes, please explain:
____
____
____

Any other observations or comments?
____
____
____

NAME_______________________________________

Any current health complaints? YES   NO

Please
expain:____
____
____
____

What Chakra(s) do these ailments correspond to?
____
____
____

What the client feels during the session?
____
____
____
____

How the client feels after the session?
____
____
____

Did you have any problems or questions while performing this session?   YES   NO
If yes, please explain:
____
____
____
____

Any other observations or comments?
____
____
____

CASE STUDY #3 DISTANT CHAKRA SESSION

NAME____

Any current health complaints? YES   NO

Please
expain:____
____
____
____

What Chakra(s) do these ailments correspond to?
____
____
____

What the client feels during the session?
____
____
____
____

How did the client feel after the session?
____
____
____

Did you have any problems or questions while performing this session?   YES   NO
If yes, please explain:
____
____
____
____

Any other observations or comments?
____
____
____

NAME____

Any current health complaints? YES   NO

Please
expain:____
____
____
____

What Chakra(s) do these ailments correspond to?
____
____
____

What the client feels during the session?
____
____
____
____

How did the client feel after the session?
____
____
____

Did you have any problems or questions while performing this session?   YES   NO
If yes, please explain:
____
____
____
____

Any other observations or comments?
____
____
____

FINAL EXAM

NAME AS YOU WOULD LIKE FOR IT TO APPEAR ON YOUR CERTIFICATE

____

What are the Chakras?

Explain why balance is so important.

List all 7 chakras, their colors, their location, their stone correspondence and their issues.

What are some differences in the chakra system of animals?   What is the same?

List three tools you can use to assist in performing chakra therapy.

What are the archetypes of the chakras?

Would you like your certification emailed _______ or mailed_______

If mailed, please provide mailing address here:

<u>**SUPPLEMENTAL STUDIES**</u>

Crystals and Gemstones

Many people use crystals and gems in their holistic practice. Crystals have powerful healing properties. Here are just a few examples that I have read about and tried myself. Place them on the chakras or just hold them in your hands and imagine energy flowing through them and into you or your client. Many people say that they amplify the energy. They are great to use during distance healings and meditation too. Quartz is used for any and all of the chakras. If you are interested in using crystals in your practice, you may want to supplement this course with the Crystal Therapy Course offered through our Institute.

Reiki

There are probably thousands of different forms of Reiki. Usui Reiki is the original and most popular, but after studying Usui, you may also want to experience other forms of this beautiful energy. You should know that no form of Reiki is more "powerful" than the Reiki you are currently experiencing. Every form of Reiki comes from the same Source; the difference comes in how we connect to this Source and how we choose to perceive the energy. In addition, Reiki Rays offers Karuna Ki, Lightarian, and Seichim Reiki.

Reflexology

Reflexology is the application of pressure and movement to the feet to effect corresponding parts of the body. Reflexologists know that the feet are a mirror image of the body. By applying one of several techniques and grips, a reflexologist can break up patterns of stress in other parts of the body. Reflexology is an art and science that goes well beyond foot massage. It is based on psychological and neurological studies.

Aromatherapy

Aromatherapy is the study of how scents affect mood and induce healing. This is perhaps the best course to supplement all other holistic therapies with, as you do not even need to anoint oils on the client for them to begin to feel the benefits. Essential oils can be applied "neat" (directly onto the feet), rubbed onto your hands, or diffused in the air.

Certification Programs, Diplomas, and Degrees

We offer certification in holistic health, spiritual health, holistic pet specialist, and angel therapy as well as a myriad of individual courses at Reiki Rays www.reikiraysinstitute.com   and Metaphysical studies at www.worldmeta.org

<u>Conclusion</u>

It has been my honor to share this course with you. I hope that while your studies may be complete that we continue to work together as you progress in your work.   Remember if you haven't done so, to schedule your chakra balancing appointment that you are entitled to with this course.

Congratulations on completing this course!

Please email case studies, exercises, and exam to: <u>reikirays@yahoo.com</u> (progress tests are yours to keep)

www.ingramcontent.com/pod-product-compliance
Lightning Source LLC
Chambersburg PA
CBHW040138240726
48664CB00002B/527

* 9 7 8 1 9 7 7 5 8 0 4 3 6 *